SCABIES

Expert Guide To Understanding Scabies
Causes, Symptoms, Preventing, Treatment
for optimal wellness

DR. DASHIELL DANIEL

Disclaimer

This book, is intended to provide information and guidance on the subject matter and is not a substitute for professional medical advice, diagnosis, or treatment.

The author, is not a medical professional, and the content presented here is based on research, general knowledge, and expert guidance available at the time of writing.

The information in this book is provided with the understanding that the author and the publisher are not engaged in rendering medical, legal, or other professional services.

Any reliance on the information contained in this book is at the reader's own risk.

While every effort has been made to ensure the accuracy and completeness of the information presented, medical knowledge is constantly evolving, and new research may supersede the content in this book. The author and the publisher make no representations or warranties of any kind, express or implied, about the completeness, accuracy, reliability, suitability, or availability concerning the information, products, services, or related graphics contained in this book.

This book may contain references or mentions of individuals, products, websites, organizations, or other names for informational purposes only.

The author does not own or endorse any such entities mentioned in the book. Any resemblance to actual persons, living or dead, or actual events is purely coincidental.

Readers are encouraged to consult with qualified healthcare professionals for medical advice, diagnosis, and treatment tailored to their specific circumstances.

The author and the publisher disclaim any liability for any loss or risk, personal or otherwise, arising directly or indirectly from the use of the information presented in this book.

By reading this book, the reader acknowledges and agrees to the terms of this disclaimer.

"Scabies" is a book that is a valuable tool for comprehending and addressing the intricacies of this extremely common skin condition.

Being the first all-inclusive guidebook written specifically for scabies, this book is important because it carefully examines the origins and history of the condition, giving readers a framework for understanding it. The first chapter clarifies how important it is to understand scabies, which sets the stage for a thorough investigation of its complex aspects.

The definition causes, and mechanisms of transmission of scabies are explored in detail in Chapter 1, which launches an academic exploration of the disease's complexities.

This section provides a fundamental knowledge basis by breaking down the Sarcoptic scabies mite and identifying risk factors that are related to it.

The next chapters provide a detailed analysis of the symptoms and signs of scabies, including common presentations, early warning signals, and other related skin alterations.

The diagnostic portion of the book offers insightful information on microscopic investigations, burrow inspections, and clinical evaluations. In Chapter 4, therapeutic options are methodically reviewed to provide readers with a thorough overview of all available interventions. These choices range from oral pharmaceuticals and topical scabicides to over-the-counter remedies and alternative therapies.

The concept is expanded in Chapters 5 and 6, which also explain preventative strategies and the worldwide effects of scabies on socioeconomics and public health. The careful examination of environmental controls, public health initiatives, and personal cleanliness behaviors gives the scholarly conversation a more realistic perspective.

In addition, the book addresses unique topics in Chapters 7 and 8, which appeal to a variety of audiences. It explores nosocomial transmission in hospital settings and looks at scabies in children, including its effects on Pediatrics and educational institutions.

In Chapter 8, new directions in research are examined, with an emphasis on therapy advancements and possible vaccinations.

Chapter 9 gently tackles the human side of scabies, giving coping mechanisms and insights into the emotional and psychological elements of living with this Illness. It is a sympathetic break from clinical topics. The complete book "Scabies" is a valuable resource for anybody looking for a full understanding of scabies and its many effects on society and health, in addition to being a reliable source of information for researchers and medical experts.

Overview

Throughout history, scabies—a highly infectious parasitic infection brought on by the mite Sarcoptic scabies—have posed a serious threat to public health.

 The beginnings and development of our knowledge of scabies are explored in The Background and History of Scabies. Scabies have affected people for ages, according to historical documents, with allusions extending back to ancient civilizations. The Latin origins of the word "scabies" emphasize how widespread this infestation is. Ancient Greek and Roman medical texts provide early accounts of scabies symptoms, illustrating the disease's persistent effect on human communities. The historical background clarifies the difficulties communities confront in combating scabies and emphasizes the significance of further study to lessen its effects.

Understanding Scabies Is Crucial

The fact that scabies is so common and affects both individuals and communities highlight how important it is to understand the problem.

Scabies affects many different demographic groups worldwide and is not only a bothersome condition. It is a serious health concern. Developing successful preventative and control methods requires an understanding of the social, economic, and public health consequences of scabies. Scabies have more negative effects than only the physical discomfort people feel; they frequently cause problems and subsequent infections. In addition, the disease's higher healthcare expenses and accompanying lost productivity demonstrate the socioeconomic impact of scabies. Therefore, to provide focused therapies and enhance overall health outcomes, healthcare practitioners, legislators, and researchers must have a thorough understanding of scabies.

Scabies's Clinical Presentation

A variety of signs and symptoms are included in the clinical presentation of scabies, which adds to the difficulty of identifying and treating the illness. Severe itching, especially at night, is the telltale indication of scabies because the mites burrow into the skin to deposit their eggs. This irritation is frequently accompanied by a rash that looks like little red papules and vesicles. Lesions are seen in many body locations such as elbows, wrists, and interdigital spaces, and their distribution varies depending on the age group. Scabies can show differently in immunocompromised persons, resulting in crusted or Norwegian scabies, and in babies, where it appears as pustules. Comprehending the many clinical manifestations is crucial for precise diagnosis and prompt commencement of suitable therapy, averting further problems and their spread.

Incidence Of Scabies

The study of scabies incidence, prevalence, and dispersion among communities is known as scabies epidemiology. Scabies are a worldwide health concern that affects people on all continents, although it is more common in places with few resources and dense populations. Scabies are spread by intimate human contact, and their persistence is aided by conditions like impoverishment, crowded living conditions, and weakened immune systems. Children, the elderly, and those with compromised immune systems are high-risk categories that are more vulnerable to scabies infestations. To lower the disease's burden and stop outbreaks in susceptible groups, targeted treatments including community-wide treatment programs and the widespread administration of drugs must be implemented with an awareness of scabies epidemiology.

The Pathogenesis Of Scabies

Clarifying the processes by which the Sarcoptic scabies mite causes harm and initiates the host's immunological response is the goal of the pathophysiology of scabies. The mite excretes its eggs and waste products in tunnels it burrows into the epidermis. When the host's immune system detects the mite, it triggers an inflammatory reaction that exacerbates the symptoms of scabies, including redness and itching. Creating focused treatment approaches requires an understanding of the molecular and cellular connections between the mite and the host. Thanks to developments in molecular biology, scientists have been able to investigate the genetic composition of Sarcoptes scabies, which has led to the discovery of possible targets for drugs and vaccine development. To improve treatment options and our capacity to control and manage scabies, a thorough understanding of the pathophysiological mechanisms underlying the illness is crucial.

Identification And Differential Identification Of Scabies

To differentiate scabies from other dermatological disorders, a comprehensive clinical assessment and analysis of many variables are necessary for the diagnosis and differential diagnosis of scabies. Although the distinctive rash and burrows may be visible in typical instances, a diagnosis might be difficult to make due to unusual presentations and variances in symptomatology. Confirmation of scabies is mostly dependent on dermatological exams, microscopic analysis of skin scrapings, and more recently, molecular diagnostic methods. In differential diagnosis, other skin disorders including eczema, insect bites, and different kinds of dermatitis are ruled out as potential mimics of scabies. Accurately diagnosing scabies is essential for starting timely and efficient treatment, avoiding drug overuse, and averting the possible negative effects of misdiagnosis.

Methods Of Scabies Treatment

Scabies treatment modalities include a variety of therapeutic treatments targeted at symptom relief, mite elimination, and prevention of reinfestation. ivermectin and permethrin are two typical topical scabicide medicines used to treat scabies infestations.

Age, whether or not a woman is pregnant, and the extent of the infestation all influence the treatment option.

To stop reinfestation, environmental precautions including cleaning clothes and bedding are also crucial. Resistance to widely prescribed drugs is a challenge in the treatment of scabies, particularly in some geographical areas. The goals of the ongoing study are to understand the processes of resistance and to discover alternate therapeutic alternatives. Healthcare professionals must have a thorough awareness of current research initiatives and treatment options to give patients high-quality care and stop the spread of scabies.

Scabies Prevention And Control Techniques

Scabies prevention and control strategies include a multimodal approach that addresses issues at the individual and community levels. To increase public understanding of the symptoms, prevention methods, and transmission of scabies, health education is essential. The three major strategies for preventing scabies infestations are good personal hygiene, appropriate sanitation, and upholding a clean living environment.

Treatment initiatives that are available to the whole community, particularly in high-risk areas, help lessen the general prevalence of scabies and break the cycle of transmission. Research is now underway to develop and apply vaccinations against scabies, which might provide long-term solutions for the control of the illness.

Effective scabies prevention and control measures require cooperation between medical experts, public health organizations, and community people.

Scabies have historical origins that have lasted through the ages, making it a major worldwide health concern today. Addressing the complexity of this parasite infestation requires an understanding of the history, clinical presentation, epidemiology, pathophysiology, diagnosis, treatment methods, and preventative measures. It is impossible to overestimate the significance of continuing research initiatives as they advance preventative care, new treatment alternatives, and improved diagnostic techniques. The combined efforts of academics, politicians, and healthcare professionals are crucial to lessening the impact of this parasite infection on people and communities throughout the world as we continue to expand our understanding of scabies.

CHAPTER ONE
COMPREHENDING SCABIES

The Sarcoptes scabies mite is the source of the extremely infectious skin condition known as scabies, which affects millions of people worldwide each year. The ailment presents as a severe, itchy rash that is frequently worse at night, placing a heavy strain on the affected communities.

It's important to learn about the definition, overview, causes, transmission, the Sarcoptes scabies mite, routes of transmission, and related risk factors to fully understand the complexities of scabies.

Definition And Synopsis

The tiny mite Sarcoptes scabiei is the cause of scabies, a parasitic infection of the skin.

The development of tunnels beneath the skin's surface, where the female mites deposit their eggs, is a defining feature of the illness.

These burrows frequently result in the appearance of a characteristic rash, which is usually accompanied by intense itching. Scabies is a disease that knows no geographical bounds; it affects people of all ages and economic statuses. Scabies cause excruciating pruritus, which can cause sleep disorders, secondary bacterial infections, and a reduction in the quality of life for individuals who have it.

Reasons And Mode Of Transmission

The Sarcoptes scabies mite, a tiny arachnid that prefers human hosts, is the main cause of scabies infestations. The symptoms of scabies are caused by mites that burrow into the epidermis, where they multiply and lay eggs. Through prolonged, direct skin-to-skin contact with an infected person, scabies can be spread. It is crucial to remember that scabies may afflict people of all socioeconomic classes and cleanliness levels; it is not just a disease of bad hygiene.

Mite Sarcoptes Scabies

The scabies mite, or Sarcoptes scabies mite, is a parasitic arthropod that only infects people.

The tiny female mites, measuring about 0.3 to 0.4 millimeters, tunnel into the epidermis to form chambers where they may deposit their eggs. These burrows trigger an inflammatory reaction in the skin, which leads to the scabies-specific rash and severe itching. The mite is an obligatory human parasite as it spends its whole life cycle on humans. Comprehending the biology and behavior of the Sarcoptes scabies mite is essential to formulating efficacious preventative and treatment measures.

Transmission Modes

The main way that scabies are spread is by direct, protracted skin contact with an infected individual. But in some circumstances, scabies can also spread through other means of transmission. Contaminated bedding, clothes, or other personal belongings that have come into touch with an infected person might cause indirect transmission. Furthermore, living arrangements that are packed, such as those seen in homes or public places, might hasten the spread of scabies. It is vital to comprehend the many pathways of transmission to execute preemptive steps and manage epidemics.

Hazard Contributors

People are more vulnerable to a scabies infestation due to several risk factors.

Close contact with an infected individual raises the risk of transmission, particularly in restricted or crowded areas. Age and gender are two demographic variables that may possibly affect vulnerability. Scabies frequently strike younger people and the elderly, as well as those with weakened immune systems. Furthermore, socioeconomic variables including living circumstances and poverty may contribute to the occurrence of scabies. To manage scabies outbreaks, public health initiatives, and tailored treatments must take these risk factors into account.

Examining the definition, overview, causes, transmission, Sarcoptes scabies mite, routes of transmission, and related risk factors is necessary to have a thorough understanding of scabies. When developing effective preventive, diagnostic, and treatment methods for scabies, healthcare providers, researchers, and policymakers need to have this multidimensional approach.

Scabies is an international health emergency that requires constant attention via research, education, and mitigation of its effects on impacted communities.

CHAPTER TWO
INDICATIONS AND SYMPTOMS

The tiny mite Sarcoptes scabiei is the source of the infectious skin condition known as scabies. It is a major worldwide public health problem due to its characteristic rash and severe itching.

Any age, gender, or socioeconomic background can contract this parasite illness, which is disseminated via intimate personal contact. Comprehending the indications and manifestations of scabies is imperative for prompt diagnosis and efficient handling.

Early Warning Indications

Scabies's early symptoms are mild and frequently missed, which makes it easier for the mites to spread. The first signs of the condition are little red pimple-like pimples on the skin.

The itching that normally goes along with these papules seems to get worse at night.

The distinctive tunnels made by the female mites are first undetectable and could be challenging to recognize without a close inspection. Since people might not be aware that they have an infestation, this is the early period when the mites are most infectious.

Typical Symptoms

Scabies can cause a variety of symptoms, but its most common symptom is itching. The itch can range in severity from minor to severe and is usually more noticeable at night, interfering with sleep and impairing the quality of life for those who experience it. The host's allergic response to the mites, their eggs, and their excrement causes the itching. In an attempt to relieve the constant itching, scratching might result in secondary bacterial infections and other problems.

Rash And Itching

Scabies are primarily characterized by itching, which is usually worst at night.

The body's immunological reaction to the mites' presence and activity on the skin causes itching. Scabies is characterized by a rash of tiny, elevated red or flesh-colored pimples. The webbed gaps between fingers, wrists, elbows, and other warm, wet parts of the body are frequently home to clusters of these bumps. As the infestation worsens, the rash may extend to other body regions, causing considerable discomfort.

Blisters And Nodules

Apart from the typical rash, nodules and blisters can also develop as a result of scabies. Nodules are hard, elevated growths that appear beneath the skin; they frequently cause localized edema. These nodules, which are a product of the host's immunological reaction, may endure long after the scabies infestation has been successfully treated. In contrast, in more severe cases, blisters may develop and may include fluid. These fluid-filled sores may be prone to burst, resulting in further difficulties, and they add to the general pain that scabies sufferers endure.

Additional Skin Changes

Other skin changes brought on by a scabies infection include redness, irritation, and excoriation from scratching. The impacted regions might have a scaly look that is similar to dermatitis or eczema. Scabies can often be misdiagnosed at first because the skin changes might be mistaken for other dermatological disorders. Burrows are the little, thread-like traces that female mites leave behind as they burrow into the skin.

This characteristic helps determine if a patient has scabies.

early intervention and successful management of this parasite infection depend on the ability to identify the telltale signs and symptoms of scabies. The typical scabies rash, itching, nodules, and other skin abnormalities all play a part in how the disease presents clinically. Not only can prompt diagnosis and treatment relieve the uncomfortable symptoms, but they also stop the infestation from spreading farther across the community. Scabies's negative effects on both people and communities at large can be reduced in large part by public health awareness and education campaigns.

CHAPTER THREE
SCABIES DIAGNOSIS

The mite Sarcoptes scabiei is the source of scabies, a highly infectious skin infection that can be difficult to diagnose because of its erratic clinical presentation. Timely response and prevention of future transmission depend on accurate identification.

Clinical Analysis

The diagnosis of scabies is based mostly on clinical examination, which entails a careful assessment of skin lesions. Dermatologists frequently concentrate on distinctive burrows, which are tiny, grayish, thread-like tracks that are usually located in the folds of the body, such as the interdigital gaps and the flexor sides of the wrists. The presence of these burrows indicates that the mite is actively tunneling beneath the skin.

Trained eyes are necessary to recognize these minor lesions, and doctors may find it helpful to visualize the lesions with a portable magnifying lens.

Examining Burrows

One essential component of the clinical examination for the diagnosis of scabies is burrow inspection. The secret to scabies infection detection lies in these burrows, which are frequently missed by the untrained eye.

The mite excavates tunnels beneath the stratum corneum, leaving behind serpiginous footprints that might be straight or curved. To identify these burrows and facilitate a timely and precise diagnosis, a methodical inspection of skin folds, interdigital areas, and genitalia is essential.

Scraping And Examining Under A Microscope

Scabies can be definitively diagnosed by scraping and microscopic investigation in addition to visual assessment. The 'Scabies Ink Test' is a method where the suspicious lesion is inked and scraped, and the material is examined under a microscope. The diagnosis is verified by the presence of fecal pellets, eggs, or mites. This approach is especially useful in situations when burrows are hidden or non-existent.

Distinctive Diagnosis

It's critical to distinguish scabies from other dermatological disorders to provide treatment appropriately. Differential diagnosis is an essential part of the diagnostic procedure since scabies and several other skin conditions share clinical characteristics.

Additional Skin Disorders

Numerous skin disorders, such as dermatitis, eczema, and insect bites, might be mistaken for scabies.

Given that erythematous, itchy papules can be a symptom of both scabies infestation and eczema, this could cause further misunderstanding. When patients appear with unusual symptoms or when scabies coexist with other skin conditions, the differential diagnosis becomes more difficult to make.

Problems With Inaccurate Diagnosis

Misdiagnosis of scabies is a prevalent problem that is exacerbated by several reasons. A diagnostic conundrum is created by the variation in clinical presentation, the symptom overlap with other skin disorders, and the possibility of atypical presentations. Furthermore, because subjective symptoms like itching can be mistaken for other dermatological or systemic illnesses, symptoms resembling scabies may be misdiagnosed.

scabies diagnosis necessitates a multimodal approach that includes microscopic investigation, burrow inspection, and clinical evaluation.

The problem is that it presents clinically like a lot of other skin disorders, which makes differential diagnosis very important to understand. Misdiagnosis emphasizes the need for a thorough and precise diagnostic procedure as it can cause treatment delays and increased transmission.

CHAPTER FOUR
POSSIBLE TREATMENTS

The tiny mite Sarcoptes scabiei is the source of the extremely infectious skin infection known as scabies. Severe itching and the appearance of tiny red pimples or rashes on the skin are the main symptoms of the disorder. To reduce symptoms, avoid problems, and stop the infestation from spreading, effective treatment is essential.

This thorough discussion will cover a wide range of scabies treatment choices, such as oral drugs, over-the-counter treatments, topical scabicides like permethrin and ivermectin, and complementary and alternative therapies.

One essential component of scabies care is the use of topical scabicides. Synthetic pyrethroids like permethrin are frequently employed as first-line therapies. It works by upsetting the mites' neurological system, which results in paralysis and finally death.

The usual protocol involves covering the entire body—aside from the head and neck—with 5% permethrin lotion. After a week, this treatment is frequently repeated to target any newly born mites. Permethrin is effective in several clinical trials and is typically well-tolerated. Permethrin resistance, however, has been documented in some areas, requiring continued investigation for substitute therapeutic approaches.

The antiparasitic drug ivermectin provides an alternate method of treating scabies. When taken orally, ivermectin paralyzes and eventually kills mites by interfering with their nerve signals.

 Those who might find topical treatments difficult will benefit most from this systemic medication. Many studies have shown that ivermectin is an effective treatment, which makes it a worthwhile choice, particularly in areas where scabies infestations are common. But since ivermectin's safety hasn't been shown beyond a reasonable doubt in some populations, such as pregnant women and those with weakened immune systems, care should be used.

Another important factor in the therapy of scabies is oral medicine. Antihistamines are a possible ingredient in these drugs to reduce inflammation and itching. Antibiotics may also be used to treat open sores and secondary bacterial infections that result from scratching. The selection of oral pharmaceuticals is customized to the individual requirements of the patient, taking into account variables including the degree of symptoms, past medical records, and the existence of adverse effects.

For those looking for accessible solutions to relieve the symptoms of scabies, over-the-counter medications provide relief. These might include ointments, lotions, or creams with benzyl benzoate, crotamiton, or sulfur as a component. Although these products could alleviate symptoms, there is considerable disagreement over their ability to completely eradicate the mites. Before using over-the-counter therapies exclusively, people should see a healthcare expert since they might not be as effective as prescription drugs.

In addition to or instead of regular medical treatments, complementary and alternative therapies encompass a wide range of interventions that are not a part of traditional medical practice. Some people go at supplementary methods when it comes to scabies, such as neem oil, tea tree oil, or sulfur supplements. Although there may be anecdotal evidence in favor of certain therapies, there is frequently a dearth of robust scientific data. To make sure that complementary and alternative therapies don't lessen the efficacy of conventional scabies treatments, people should approach these treatments cautiously and speak with healthcare professionals.

Scabies treatment options are diverse and include both systemic treatments like ivermectin and topical treatments like permethrin. The holistic method of treating this parasite infection includes complementary treatments, over-the-counter drugs, and oral pharmaceuticals. The patient's preferences, the extent of the infestation, and any underlying medical concerns all play a role in the choice of an appropriate treatment plan.

The tactics for preventing scabies and enhancing patient outcomes will be further refined as research advances new therapy choices and a deeper comprehension of resistance mechanisms is developed.

CHAPTER FIVE
CONTROL AND PREVENTION

The tiny mite Sarcoptes scabiei is the source of the extremely infectious skin infection known as scabies. If left untreated, this parasite infection can cause subsequent bacterial infections and is marked by severe itching and a unique rash. Several ideas are involved in the prevention and management of scabies, including environmental interventions, public health tactics, and personal hygiene habits.

Scabies may be prevented and controlled in large part by following good personal hygiene habits. Individuals who practice proper personal cleanliness can greatly lower their chance of infestation. Mites and their eggs can be eliminated by regular, thorough body cleaning, with specific attention to the regions between fingers, wrists, elbows, and genitalia.

Using fresh, often laundered bedding and clothes also reduces the possibility of transmission.

 Furthermore, scabies cannot spread among people if personal objects like combs, clothes, and towels are not shared.

Environmental interventions have a major role in preventing scabies. Maintaining hygienic and clean-living areas is essential to preventing the spread of mites. Regularly cleaning and vacuuming the living space can aid in the removal of mites and their eggs from the surrounding area. To further help eradicate mites, wash bedding, clothes, and personal things in hot water and dry them at a high temperature. To stop the spread of infection, communal areas including schools, dorms, and medical facilities must be meticulously cleaned.

One of the most important scabies preventive strategies in the context of environmental measures is avoiding close contact. The risk of transmission can be reduced by reducing close physical contact since scabies mites transfer by direct skin-to-skin contact. Until they have finished the necessary treatment and are no longer infectious, those with suspected or confirmed scabies infestations should avoid close contact with others. It is imperative to take this preventive action to stop the spread of scabies in homes, workplaces, and communities.

Large-scale scabies prevention depends on public health initiatives. The dissemination of information on scabies, its symptoms, and preventative measures is mostly the responsibility of health authorities and institutions. Campaigns for public health can inform people about the value of maintaining a clean environment, avoiding close contact in particular situations, and maintaining good personal hygiene. It needs cooperation between legislators, community leaders, and healthcare experts to put into practice efficient scabies prevention and control measures.

Scabies prevention and control require a multimodal strategy that includes environmental controls, public health initiatives, and personal hygiene habits. People and communities may lessen the prevalence of scabies and its related consequences by advocating for and putting these ideas into practice. Sustainable attempts to manage scabies and reduce their impact on public health need education, awareness, and collaboration between communities and healthcare professionals.

CHAPTER SIX
IMPACT ON PUBLIC HEALTH

The Sarcoptes scabies mite is the source of the extremely infectious skin infection known as scabies. It causes severe skin rashes and itching, which can lead to several consequences. Comprehending the effects of scabies on public health is crucial to formulating efficacious preventative and treatment approaches.

This section will explore the global impact of scabies, looking at their frequency and effects globally.

Scabies are a serious worldwide health concern, with millions of cases recorded each year. Although the parasite infection affects people of all ages and socioeconomic backgrounds, low-resource environments are most affected.

Scabies are a common disease in poorer nations due to congested living conditions and poor access to healthcare.

The mite's capacity to move quickly throughout communities and cause epidemics that may overwhelm regional health systems adds to the burden.

Understanding the socioeconomic impact of scabies is essential to comprehend the disease's wider effects. The financial repercussions of this infestation are enormous for families, individuals, and healthcare systems. The direct and indirect expenses of managing scabies contribute to the financial burden. Medication expenditures, diagnostic test costs, and consultation fees are examples of direct costs. Indirect expenses include lost production from sick days, decreased ability to work, and permanent disability from severe scabies consequences.

An additional aspect of the socioeconomic burden of scabies is social shame. Affected people frequently experience prejudice and exclusion from their communities. The societal shame associated with scabies is exacerbated by the condition's obvious symptoms, which include rashes and skin sores. Discrimination is further fueled by misconceptions and ignorance as individuals may have unjustified worries of spreading. The mental health of scabies sufferers is negatively impacted by this stigma, which also makes community-based preventive and control initiatives more difficult.

The financial consequences of scabies go beyond personal medical bills and have an effect on society as a whole. Communities with high rates of scabies prevalence see lower worker productivity and higher healthcare costs. The financial impact is especially noticeable in underdeveloped areas, where the expenses of controlling scabies epidemics can put further strain on already precarious healthcare infrastructure. Scabies can also have long-term effects that, if ignored, can result in chronic problems that worsen the disease's effects on afflicted people and their communities economically.

The social stigma attached to scabies stems from ingrained cultural beliefs and misconceptions regarding the illness. Because the skin sores are visible, people with scabies may experience prejudice and social isolation. The psychological pain that stigmatization may cause can exacerbate the burden on those who are plagued by mental illness. A common cause of social disengagement is the fear of being branded as dirty or infectious, which can damage connections with others and impede one's ability to further one's education or career. To encourage early discovery, prompt medical attention, and community support for scabies victims, it is imperative to address societal stigma.

In conclusion, millions of people worldwide suffer from scabies, a disease that is especially prevalent in areas with inadequate resources. Scabies have a complex socioeconomic impact that includes financial losses, lost production, and social shame. Comprehending these aspects is essential for formulating all-encompassing public health approaches targeted at scabies prevention, early identification, and efficient care. Together, we can reduce the worldwide burden of scabies by working toward destigmatization campaigns, better healthcare access, and community education to lessen the disease's far-reaching effects.

CHAPTER SEVEN
SPECIAL CONSIDERATIONS

The Sarcoptes scabies mite, which burrows into the skin and causes an excruciatingly painful rash, is the culprit behind the scabies infection. Regarding scabies, special concerns include several factors, such as how the disease manifests in particular groups and environments.

The effects of scabies on children are an important topic to research. Scabies pose particular difficulties and factors to take into account in pediatric instances. Scabies in children might present with unique clinical signs, thus it's important to give special consideration to the diagnosis and treatment of this population. Furthermore, scabies control in childcare centers and schools is a crucial issue that requires extra attention. Because these surroundings are communal in nature, there is a risk of quick transmission, thus it is important to have a thorough grasp of preventative measures and efficient intervention procedures.

Because children have a distinct demography, scabies in children, also known as pediatric scabies, require specialist care.

Children often have unusual symptoms, which makes diagnosis difficult. Scabies are characterized by a pruritic rash, which might show differently in children and can result in a misdiagnosis or a delay in starting therapy. Age-appropriate medicine and possible immune system development difficulties are important factors to take into account while managing pediatric scabies. Furthermore, it is important to carefully assess how scabies affect children's psychological well-being, including any possibility for stigmatization.

Because of the close closeness of persons at schools and daycares, these environments have the potential to be hotspots for the spread of scabies.

Play areas and schools are social spaces, which increases the likelihood of scabies spreading quickly among kids. Scabies control in schools and childcare centers requires a multimodal strategy that includes early case detection, parent communication, and preventative measure execution. To provide a supportive atmosphere for prompt intervention and lower the likelihood of outbreaks, staff, parents, and caregivers must receive education about scabies signs and prevention measures.

Extending beyond the pediatric domain, scabies inside hospital environments are an additional aspect that needs particular attention.

There is a risk of nosocomial scabies transmission, especially in nursing homes and hospitals.

Scabies outbreaks linked to healthcare facilities might provide difficulties because of the susceptibility of patients and the possibility of mite transmission among medical personnel. Ensuring that hospital facilities are free from scabies outbreaks requires strong infection control protocols. This entails the prompt detection of instances, segregation of impacted persons, and rigorous adherence to hygienic protocols by medical staff.

The complicated problem of nosocomial scabies transmission in hospital environments is impacted by several variables, including patient mobility, shared medical equipment, and the frequency of underlying medical disorders. Apart from the difficulties associated with identifying and treating scabies in medical environments, stopping their spread in these settings calls a concerted effort.

To effectively manage scabies in hospitals and other healthcare institutions, strict infection control procedures, frequent observation, and education of healthcare personnel are essential.

Infection control strategies are essential for reducing the spread of scabies in medical environments. It is crucial to follow procedures precisely, which include decontaminating the surroundings, wearing personal protective equipment, and practicing good hand hygiene. To stop outbreaks and take prompt action, healthcare providers must be alert in identifying scabies signs, especially in high-risk groups. Effective strategies for scabies prevention within hospital environments are established and maintained via the joint efforts of infection control practitioners, administrative personnel, and healthcare teams.

particular issues concerning scabies include a variety of aspects, such as the distinct ways in which the infestation presents itself in youngsters and the difficulties that arise from its existence in medical environments. Effective scabies prevention, diagnosis, and management in a variety of locations and groups depends on an understanding of these factors. Targeted methods that lessen the risk of transmission and lessen the burden of scabies can be implemented in various environments by adapting techniques to the unique needs of children, schools, and healthcare facilities.

CHAPTER EIGHT
EMERGING TRENDS AND RESEARCH

The extremely infectious skin infection known as scabies, which is brought on by the parasitic mite Sarcoptic scabies, has been a major global public health problem. Over time, the knowledge and treatment of scabies have changed as a result of continuous study on many facets of the illness. This section delves into the recent developments and research surrounding scabies, looking at current projects, prospective vaccinations, and therapeutic advancements.

Current Research

Researchers studying scabies are working to better understand the parasite, its life cycle, and the intricate host-parasite interactions, that keep the field vibrant and ever-evolving.

Current research projects are diverse and include pathophysiology, epidemiology, diagnosis, and the creation of new treatment modalities.

To clarify the genetic and molecular processes behind the pathogenicity of the mite and the host's immunological response, researchers are carrying out several in-depth investigations.

Furthermore, epidemiological studies are crucial for determining risk factors, mapping the worldwide incidence of scabies, and comprehending the dynamics of outbreaks. These initiatives provide important data for focused control strategy development and public health measures.

To provide insight into the larger context of this neglected tropical illness, ongoing research also examines the socioeconomic aspects that may contribute to the persistence and spread of scabies.

It is essential to comprehend the pathophysiology of scabies to create successful therapies. Researchers are looking at the immune reactions that the mite causes as well as the strategies the parasite uses to get past the host's defenses.

This information is crucial for developing treatment plans that improve treatment results by regulating the host immune system in addition to getting rid of the mite.

Possible Immunizations

One potentially effective approach to scabies control is vaccination. The goal is to create vaccines that can provide protection against infestations of Sarcoptes scabiei. Although there are obstacles due to the intricacy of the human immune response and the mite's life cycle, research is making great progress in identifying viable vaccine candidates.

Targeting important antigens that the mite expresses at different phases of its life cycle is one strategy. A vaccination could stop scabies infestations from starting or lessen the severity of symptoms by stimulating the immune system against these antigens. Furthermore, to improve the specificity and effectiveness of prospective vaccinations, researchers are investigating the use of recombinant antigens.

When creating a vaccination against scabies, the target population—which includes susceptible populations like children and those with weakened immune systems—must also be taken into account. To evaluate a proposed vaccine's safety, immunogenicity, and protective effectiveness, clinical studies are necessary. Research institutes, pharmaceutical firms, and public health organizations must work together to advance vaccine development and guarantee that vaccines are available to communities that are at risk.

Improvements In Medical Care

Scabies treatment methods have advanced significantly, with the goals of achieving more effectiveness, fewer side effects, and easier administration.

Topical acaricides like ivermectin and permethrin are still essential therapies, but new formulations and delivery systems are being investigated to maximize their efficacy.

The creation of substitute topical medications with better safety profiles and lower environmental effects is one area of advancement.

 Examining novel formulations and delivery methods guarantees the availability of a range of treatment alternatives and helps address issues like resistance to conventional acaricides. Furthermore, studies are being conducted to improve treatment plans, taking into account variables like the length of therapy and the necessity of recurrent treatments to achieve total eradication.

Systemic therapies have become more popular because of their effectiveness and ease, especially oral ivermectin. To enhance therapy results, ongoing research aims to evaluate long-term safety, optimize dosing schedules, and investigate possible combination treatments.

Another field of study that supports the monitoring of therapy efficacy and informs decisions about treatment length and follow-up is the development of biomarkers for treatment response.

Investigations are also being conducted into complementary methods, such as the use of adjuvant treatments and the research of host-directed interventions. Immunomodulatory drugs may strengthen the host's defenses naturally while lessening the scabies-related inflammatory response, according to research.

These developments underline the significance of ongoing research to address current issues and enhance patient outcomes by adding to the wide and dynamic landscape of scabies treatment choices.

the continuous investigation into scabies demonstrates a multifaceted endeavor to decipher the intricacies of this parasite disease.

The scientific community is actively working to advance our knowledge and resources for managing and preventing scabies, from comprehending the basic biology of the mite to creating novel treatment modalities and investigating immunization approaches. These initiatives have the potential to lessen the impact of this neglected tropical illness on global health in addition to advancing our knowledge of scabies.

CHAPTER NINE
SCABIOUS LIVING

People who have scabies may find it difficult and upsetting to live with this infectious skin infection. The tiny mite Sarcoptes scabies, which burrow into the skin and cause excruciating itching and agony, are the cause of scabies. Because of the stigma attached to the illness, emotional and psychological stress frequently accompany physical symptoms. Since the infestation spreads through intimate contact, it poses a serious risk to public health in several contexts, including crowded housing, institutions, and medical facilities.

The constant itching, which might be worse at night, is one of the main difficulties of having scabies. The constant scratching raises the possibility of subsequent bacterial infections by causing open sores. The noticeable skin rash and lesions can lower someone's quality of life by making them feel embarrassed and self-conscious. Scabies are extremely contagious, which further increases worries about spreading to friends, relatives, or coworkers. This can cause social isolation and damaged relationships.

Adaptive Techniques:

Scabies require a multimodal approach to treatment that takes care of the infestation's psychological effects in addition to its physical symptoms. To eradicate the mites and their eggs, topical treatments such as scabicide creams or lotions are frequently administered.

Nonetheless, the recuperation procedure can need some time, and throughout this time, people want efficient coping mechanisms to handle their bodily unease and psychological turmoil.

Keeping up with hygiene is one coping mechanism to stop scabies from spreading to other people and reduce the chance of developing secondary infections.

Bedding, clothes, and personal belongings can be regularly washed in hot water to get rid of mites and lower the risk of re-infestation. Additionally, keeping the afflicted regions clean and refraining from scratching might hasten recovery and minimize problems

Aspects Of Emotion And Psychology:

Although they are sometimes disregarded, the emotional and psychological effects of having scabies are vital to the general well-being of those who are afflicted. Shame, embarrassment, and loneliness can result from the stigma attached to scabies. People may be afraid of other people's opinions, which makes it difficult for them to talk honestly about their illness and ask for help.

Two frequent psychological effects of scabies infection are anxiety and sadness. The constant itching and obvious skin symptoms might have a detrimental effect on one's perception of one's physique and self-worth.

The emotional strain may be exacerbated by increased anxiety brought on by the worry of spreading the mites to other people.

To offer complete and efficient care, medical professionals must address not just the physical symptoms of scabies but also its psychological and emotional components.

SUMMARY

Living with scabies is more than just enduring the physical pain brought on by the infestation. Individuals may suffer major emotional and psychological consequences that lower their general quality of life. Scabies demands a multifaceted approach to management that takes into account the mental and physical aspects of the illness.

Good coping mechanisms include following medical advice, keeping up with personal cleanliness, and reaching out for social support.

To reduce stigma, debunk myths, and educate people about scabies, healthcare practitioners are essential. Healthcare providers may promote the overall well-being of scabies patients by encouraging open communication and offering psychological assistance.

To debunk myths and encourage early identification and treatment, awareness campaigns and educational activities are essential when treating scabies on a public health level. Preventing the spread of scabies can also involve taking action to enhance living conditions in high-risk environments, such as crowded institutions.

treating scabies requires a thorough and compassionate strategy. Healthcare providers may treat scabies patients more effectively and holistically if they take into account not just the physical symptoms but also the psychological and emotional ones.

Furthermore, spreading knowledge and awareness among the community can help lessen the stigma attached to scabies and provide a welcoming atmosphere for those who are afflicted.